BEGINNERS MANDALA MEDITATION

COLORING BOOK

MANDALA'S ARE BEAUTIFUL DESIGNS THAT ARE CREATED TO VISUALLY REPRESENT THE UNIVERSE FROM AN EXTERNAL POINT OF VIEW OR CAN BE USED FOR MEDITATIONAL PURPOSES FOR AN INTERNAL USE. WE USE MANDALAS IN MEDITATION TO HELP US WORK THROUGH PROBLEMS, OR TO HELP EASE AND FOCUS THE MIND. YOU CAN STARE AT MANDALAS AND ALLOW THE DESIGN TO BECOME YOUR FOCUS IN MEDITATION. YOU CAN DRAW MANDALAS AND ALLOW YOUR ENERGY TO FOCUS NATURALLY UPON THE CREATION OF THE MANDALA. YOU CAN ALSO COLOR MANDALAS TO FOCUS YOUR DIRECTION AND ATTENTION. THIS COLORING BOOK CONTAINS SIMPLE PICTURES TO COLOR THAT CAN BE FRAMED OR HUNG ON A WALL FOR VISUAL MEDITATIONAL USE.

THIS IS A GREAT ACTIVITY FOR CHILDREN & ADULTS AS IT HELPS TO FOCUS THE MIND AND BRING YOU TO A POINT WHERE YOU CAN BEGIN TO LEARN THE BASIC CONCEPTS OF MEDITATION. THE FUN DESIGNS YOU COLOR WILL HELP THEM NATURALLY LEARN TO DEVELOP THE FOCUS NEEDED FOR MEDITATION. INCLUDED IN THE BOOK ARE SPIRITUAL PICTURES & QUOTES TO HELP DIRECT YOUR MIND AS YOU COLOR.

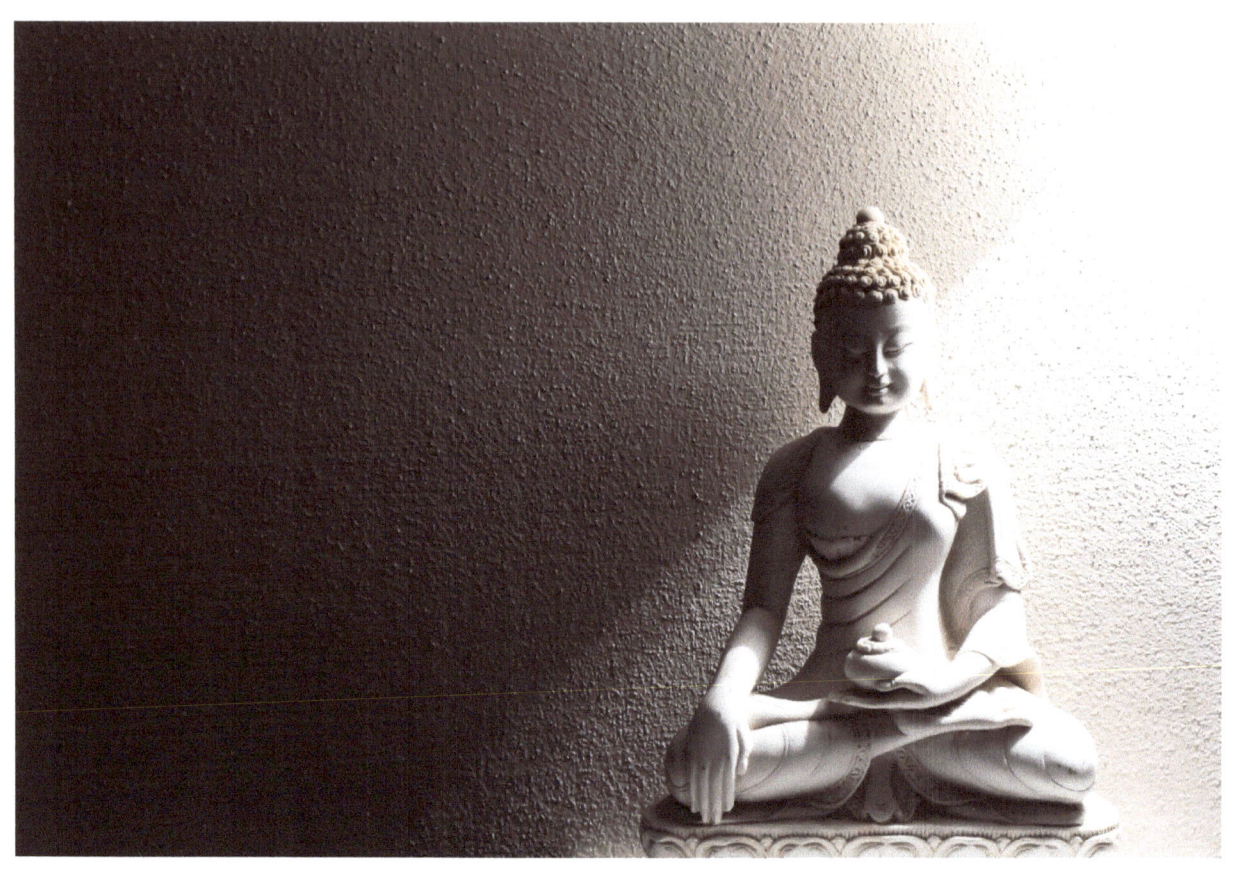

IN THE END THESE THINGS MATTER

HOW WELL DID YOU LOVE?

HOW FULLY DID YOU LIVE?

HOW DEEPLY DID YOU LET GO?

GUATAMA BUDDHA

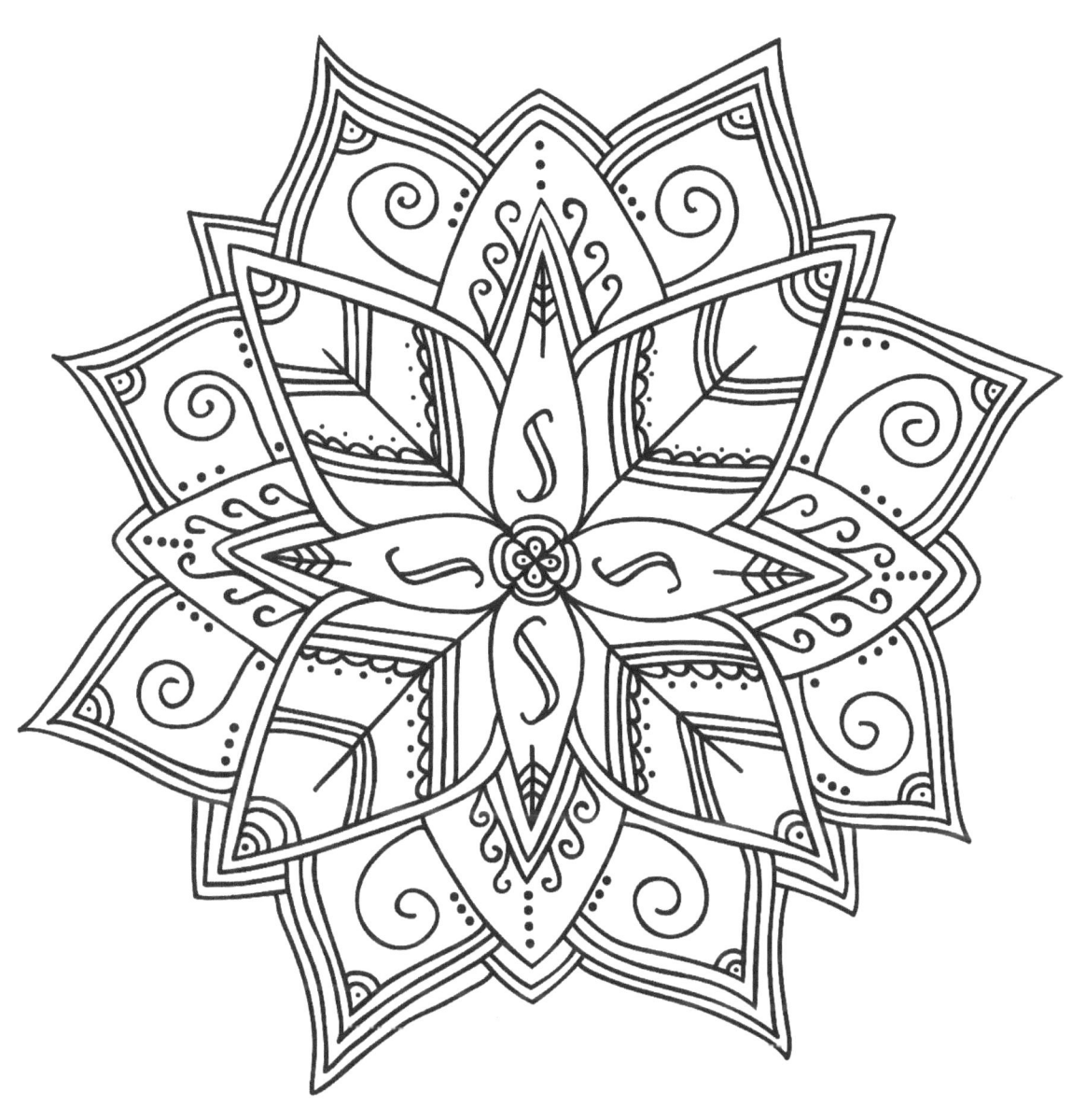

"Happiness does not depend on what you have or who you are. It solely relies on what you think."

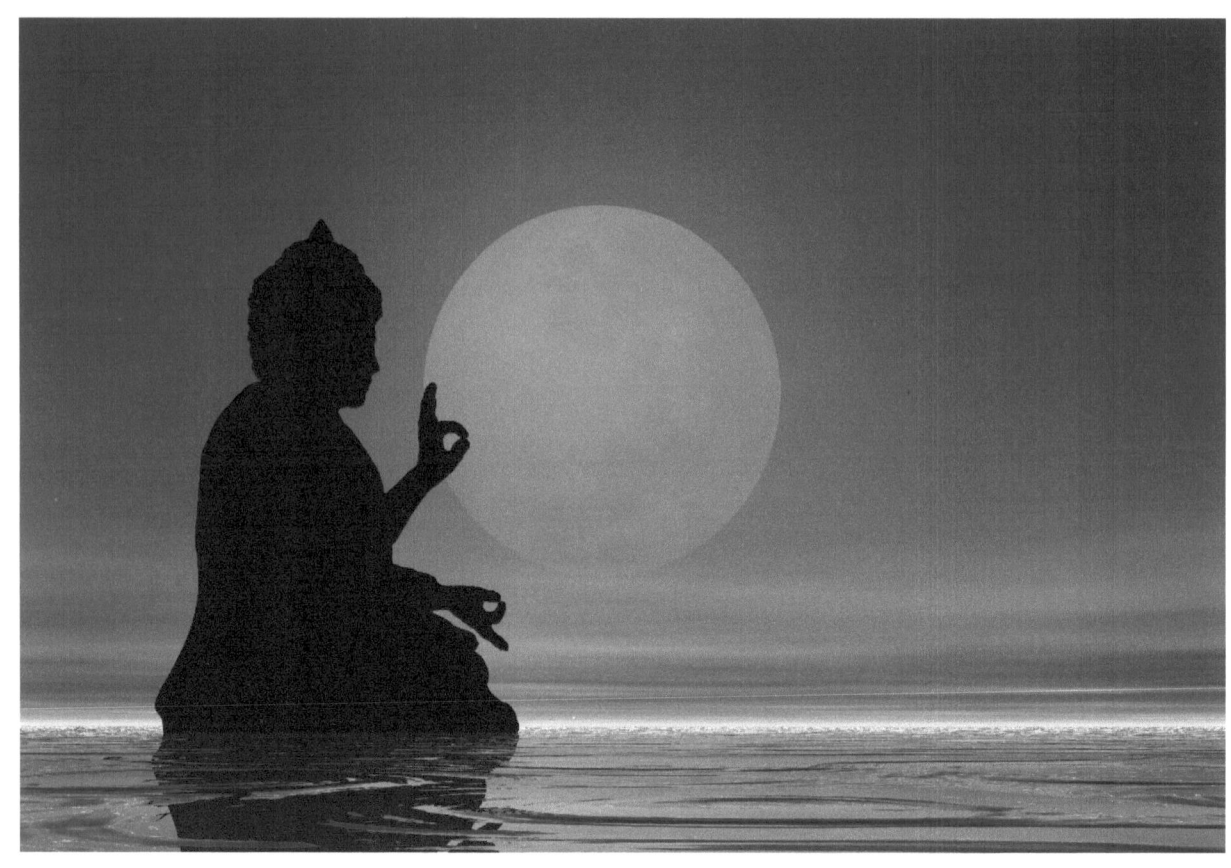

DO NOT DWELL IN THE PAST,

DO NOT DREAM OF THE FUTURE,

CONCENTRATE THE MIND

ON THE PRESENT MOMENT

BUDDHA

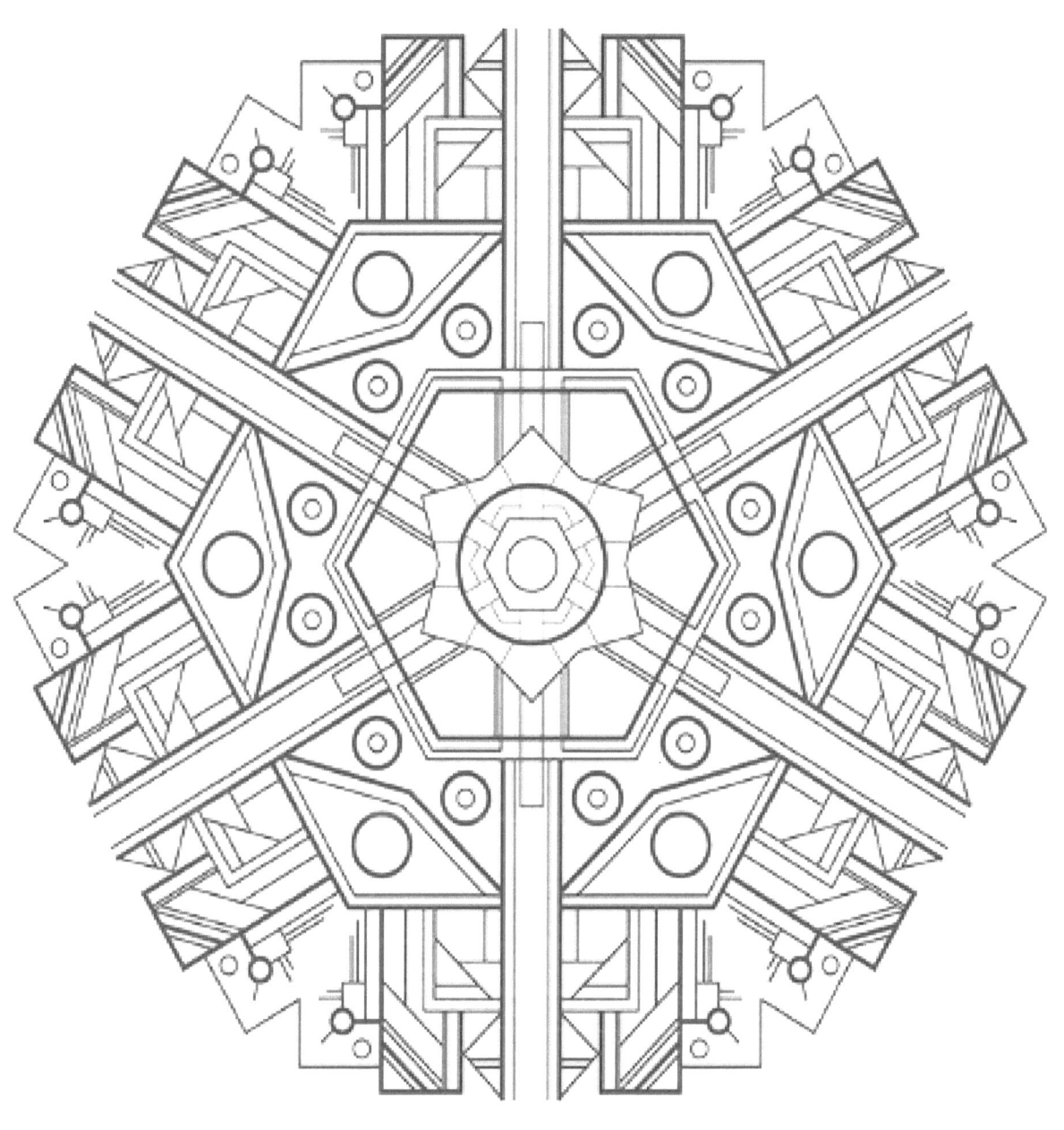

"Our greatest glory is not in never falling, but in rising every time we fall."

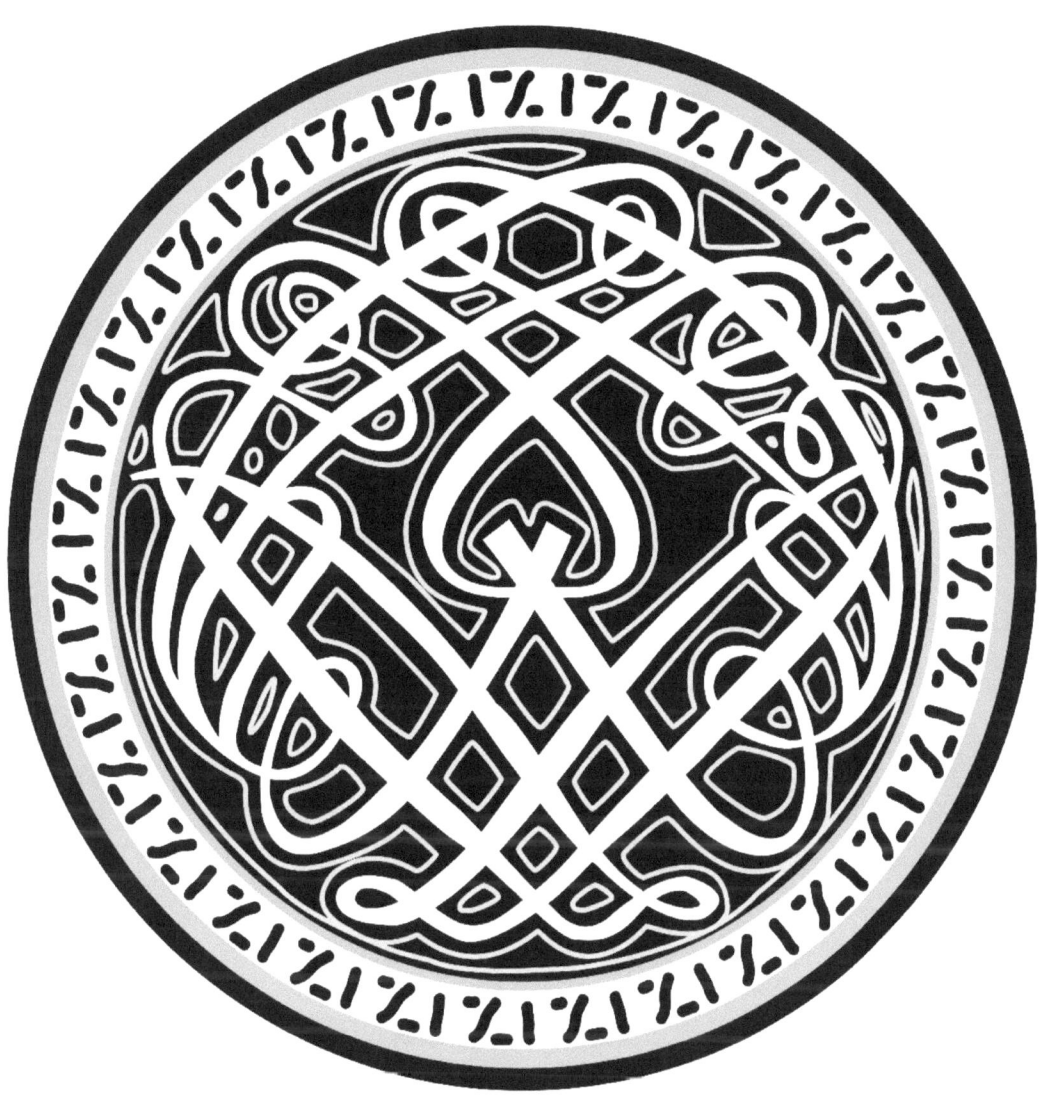

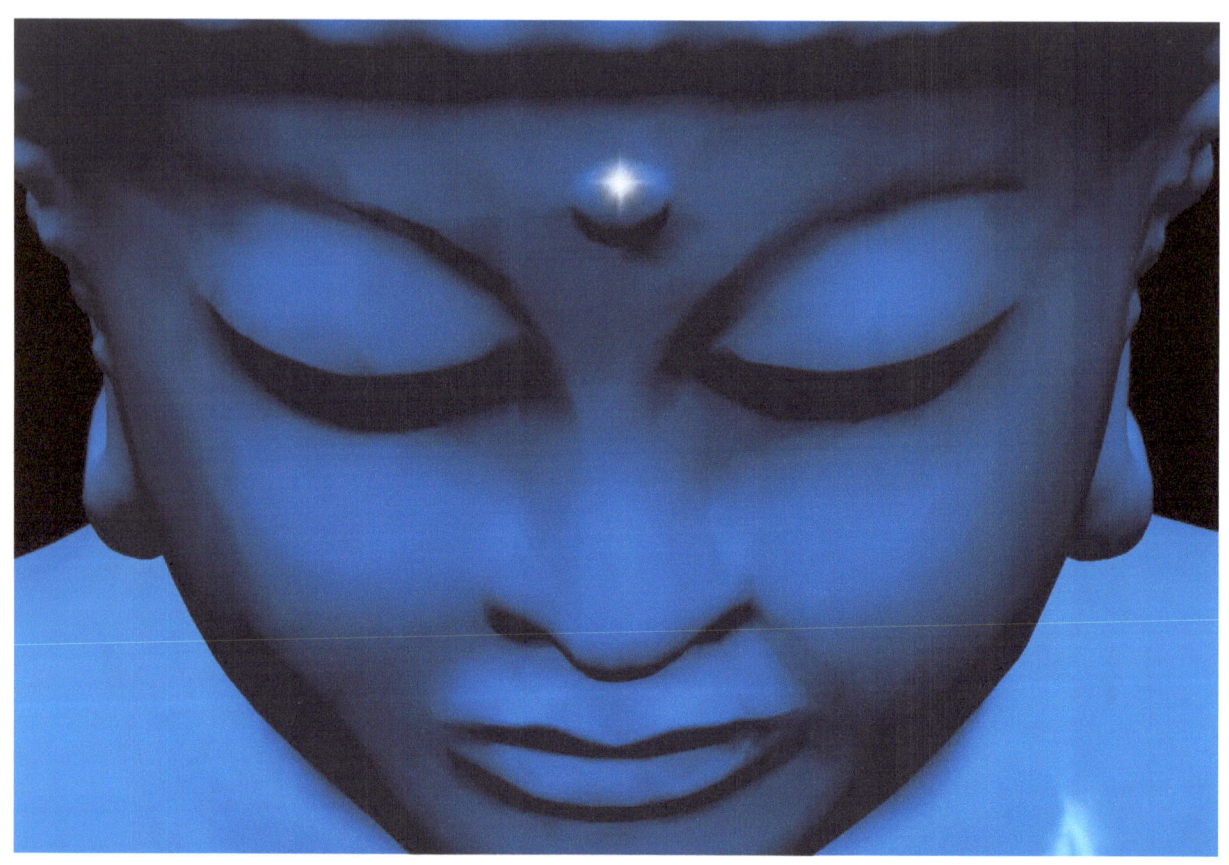

BE THE CHANGE YOU WANT

TO SEE IN THE WORLD!

MAHATMA GANDHI

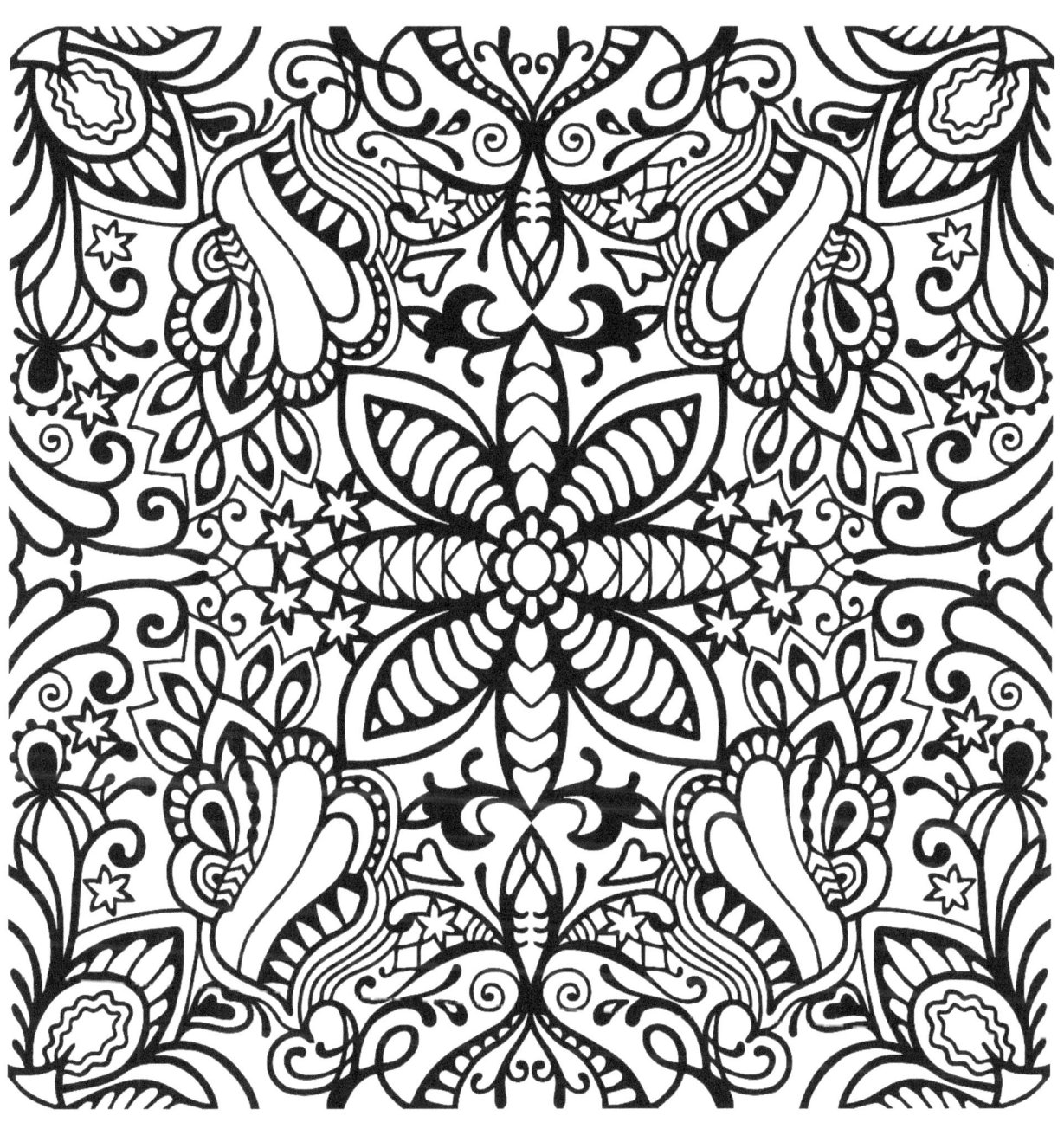

"When you are content to be simply yourself and don't compare or compete, everbody will respect you."

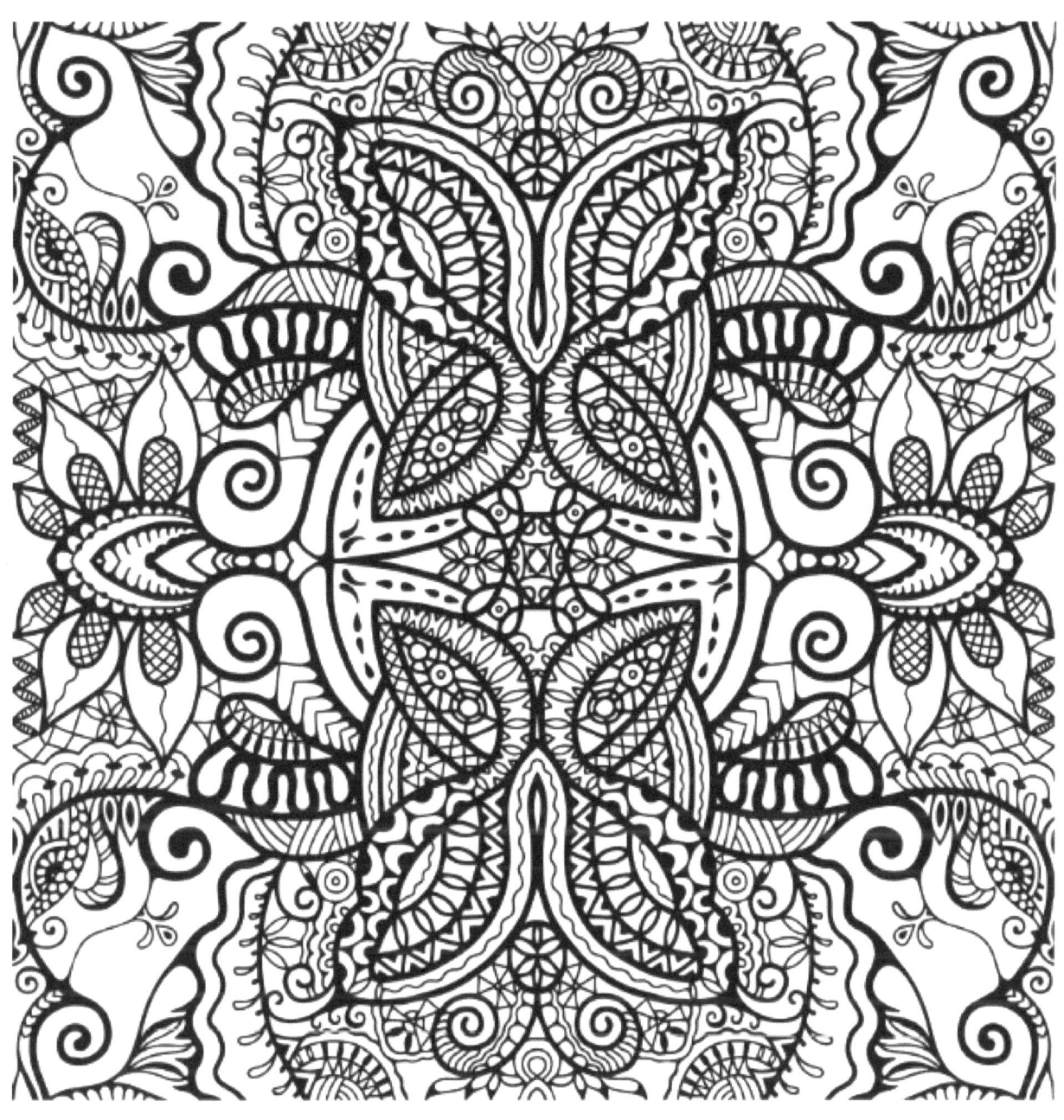

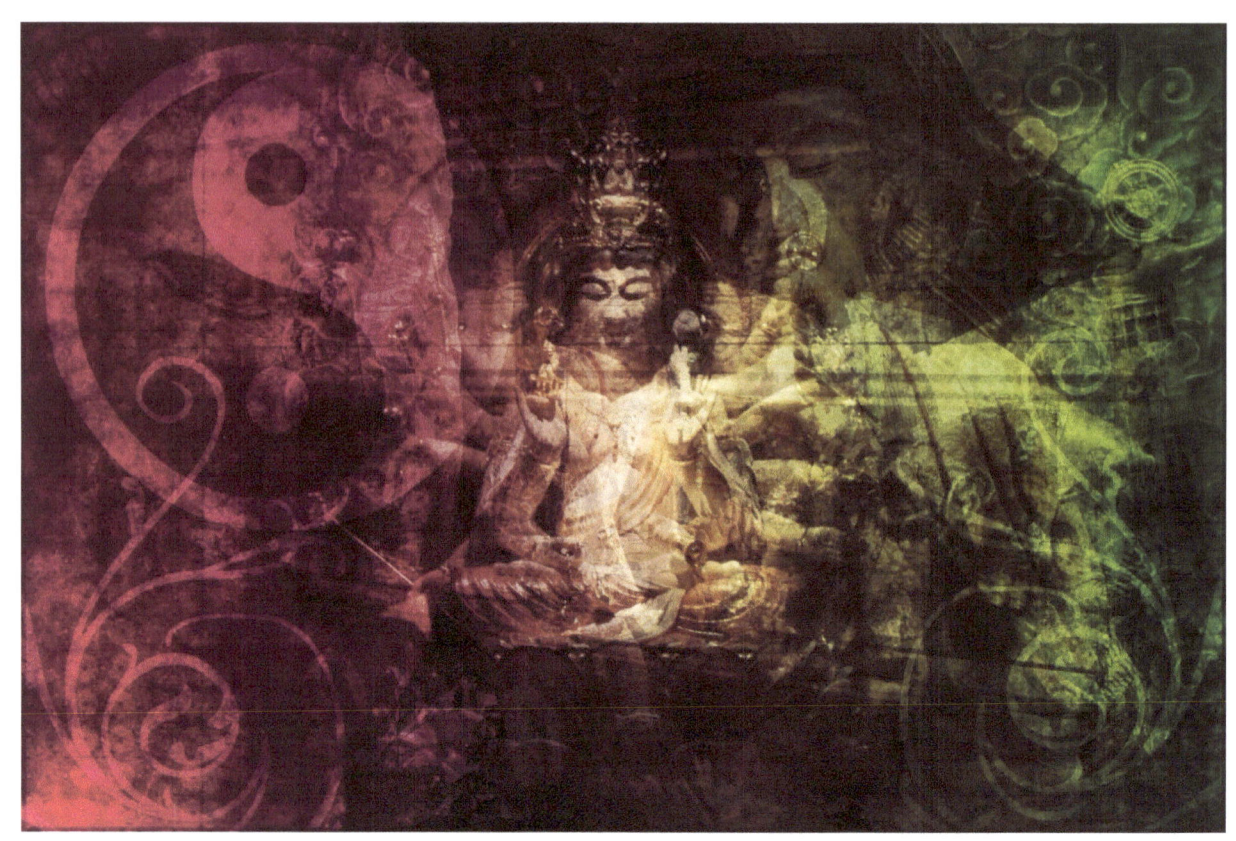

NATURE DOES NOT HURRY

YET EVERYTHING IS ACCOMPLISHED!

LAO TZU

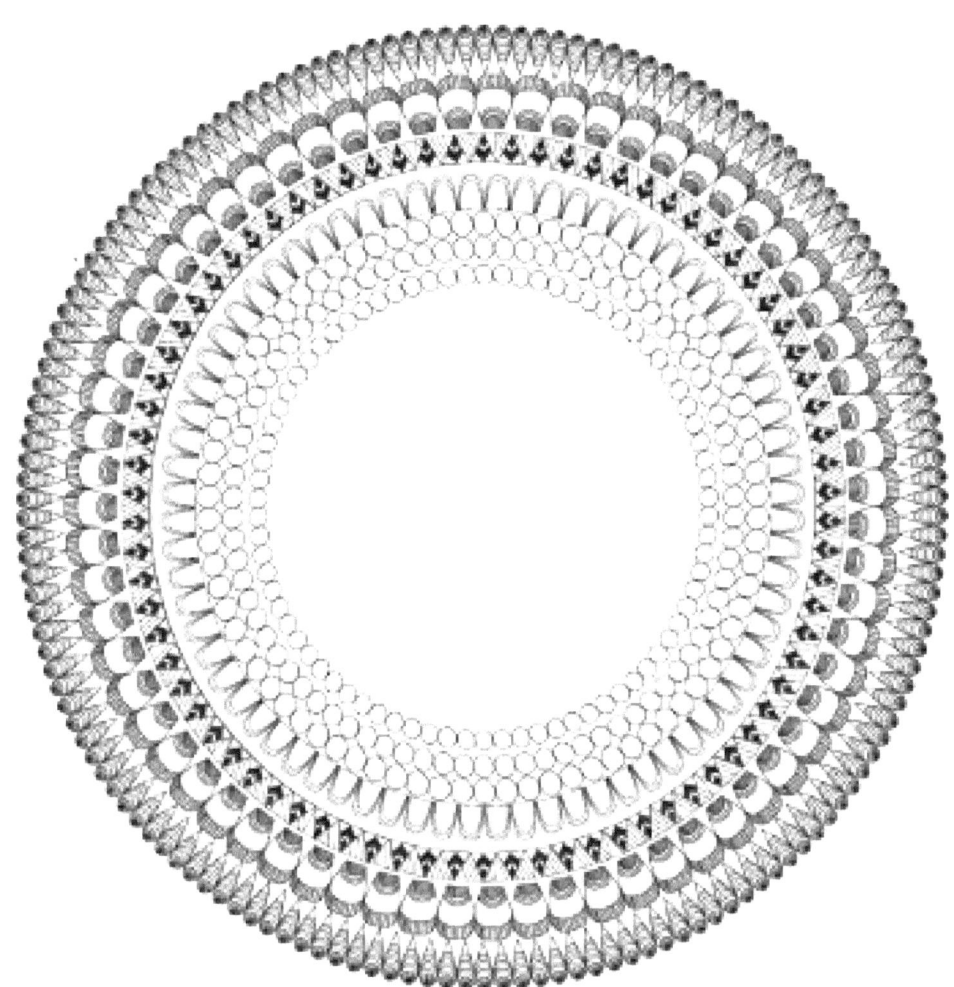

Life is short, **LIVE IT.**
Love is rare, **GRAB IT.**
Anger is bad, **DUMP IT.**
Fear is awful, **FACE IT.**
Memories are sweet,
CHERISH IT.

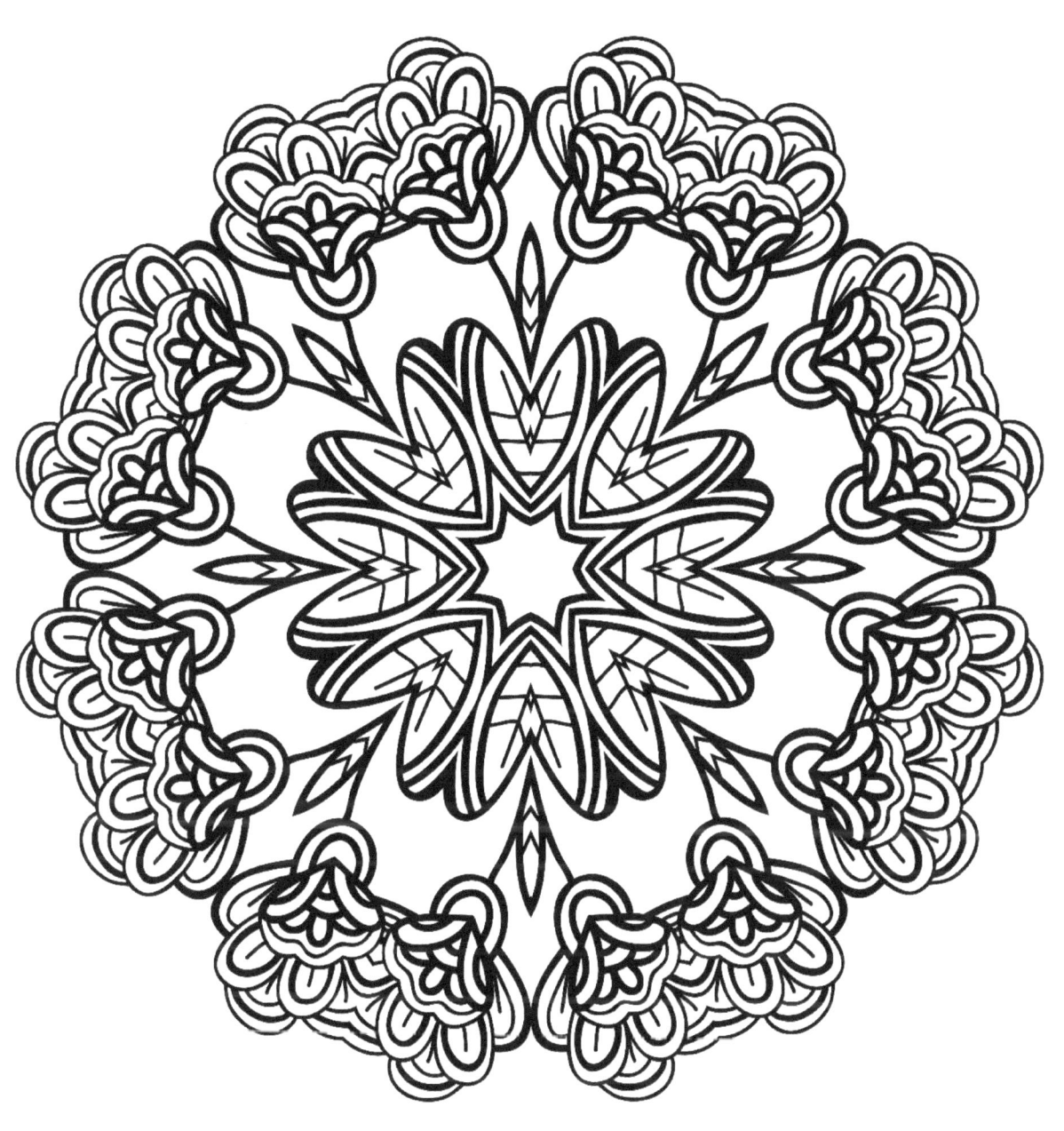

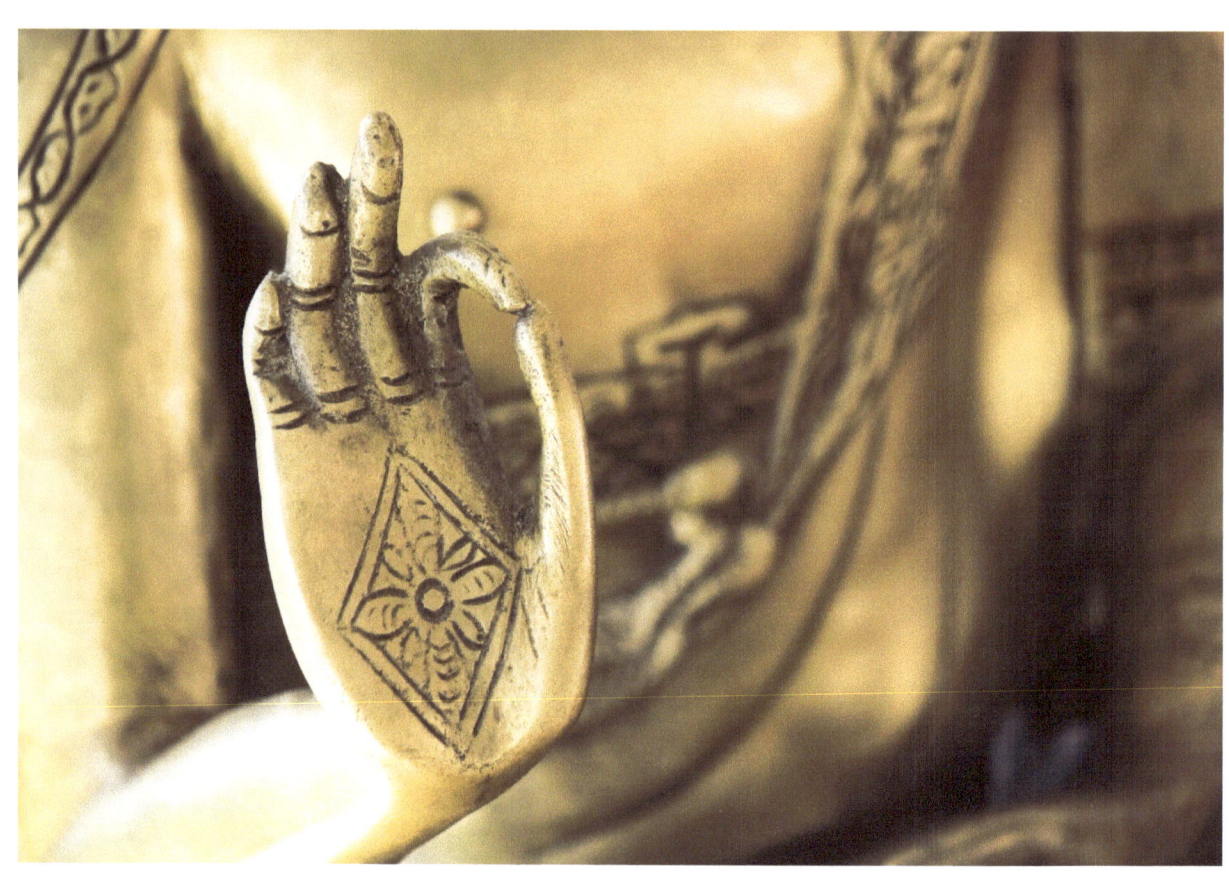

IF WE ONLY SEEK TO DESTROY

THEN WE FAIL TO CREATE!

RICE

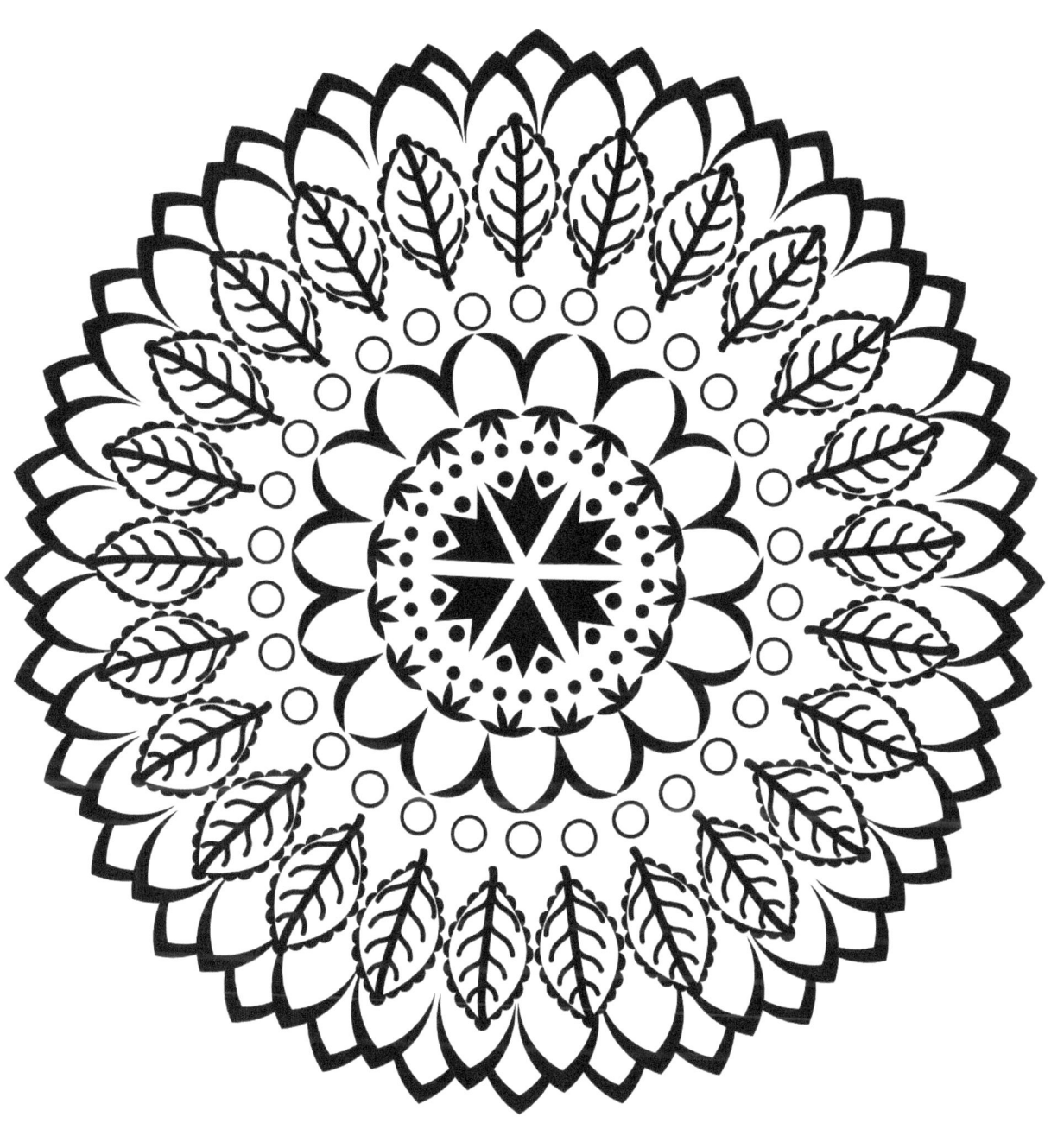

"When I let go of what I am, I become what I might be."

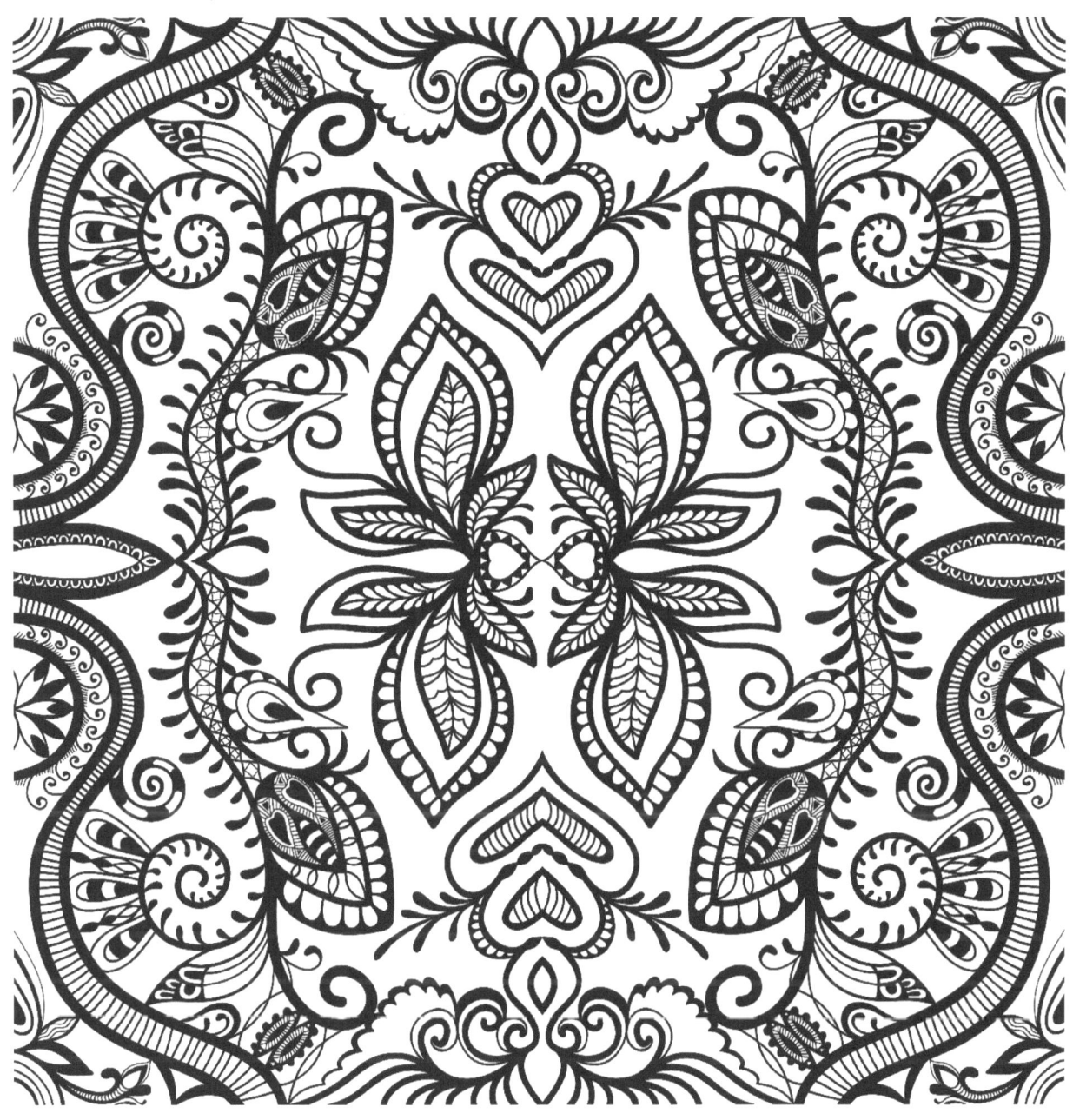

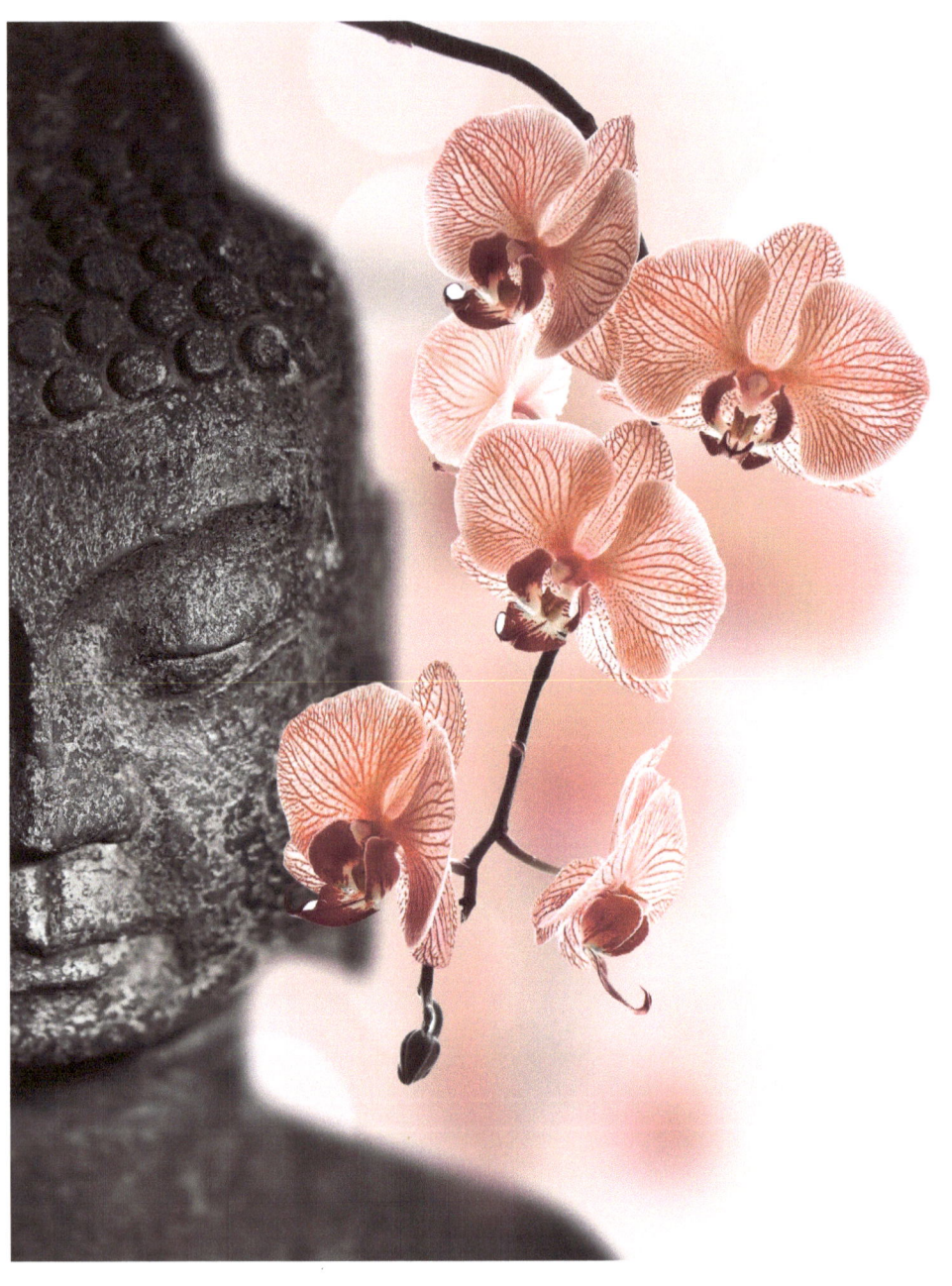

WONDER IS THE BEGINNING

OF WISDOM!

SOCRATES

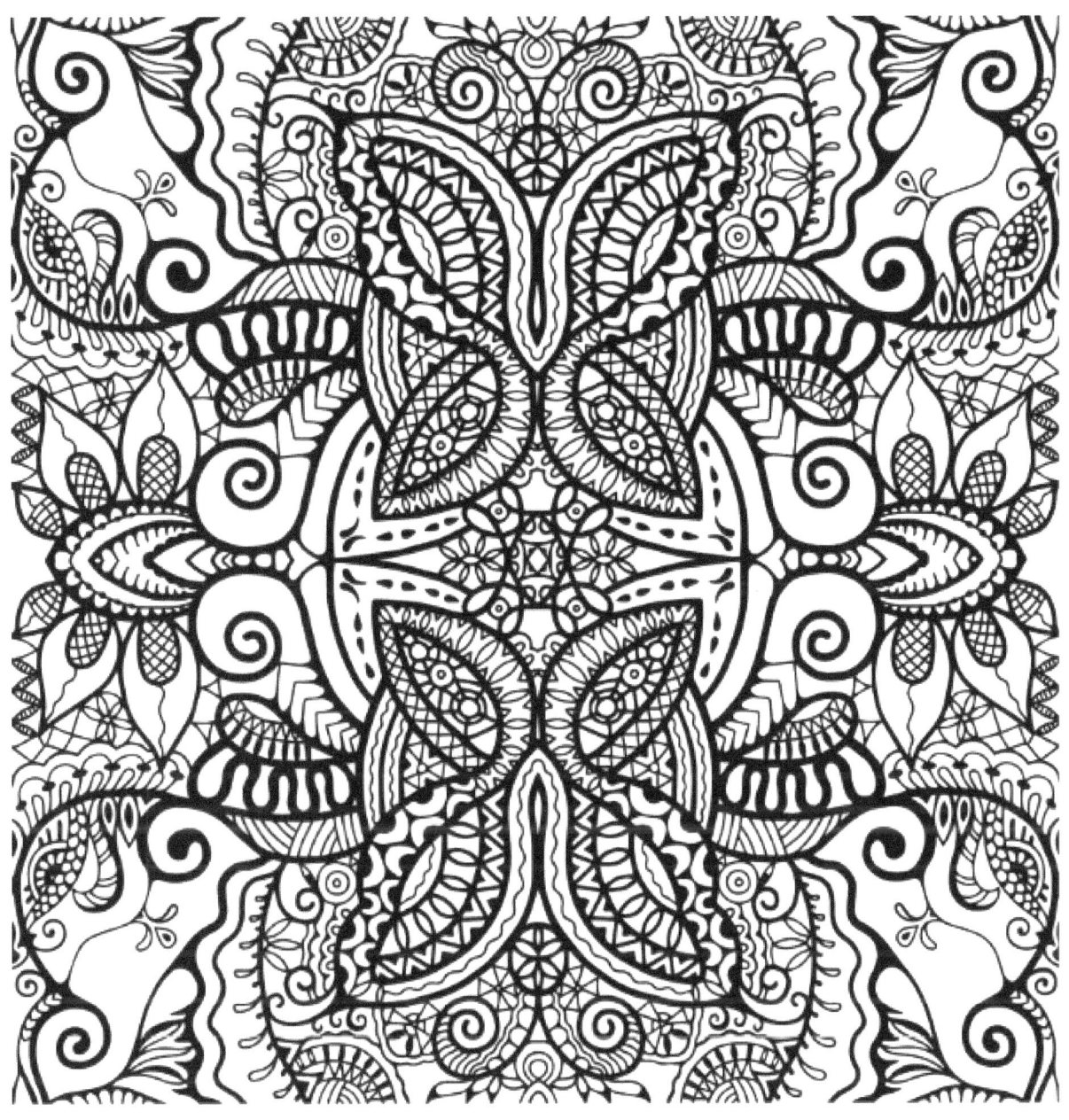

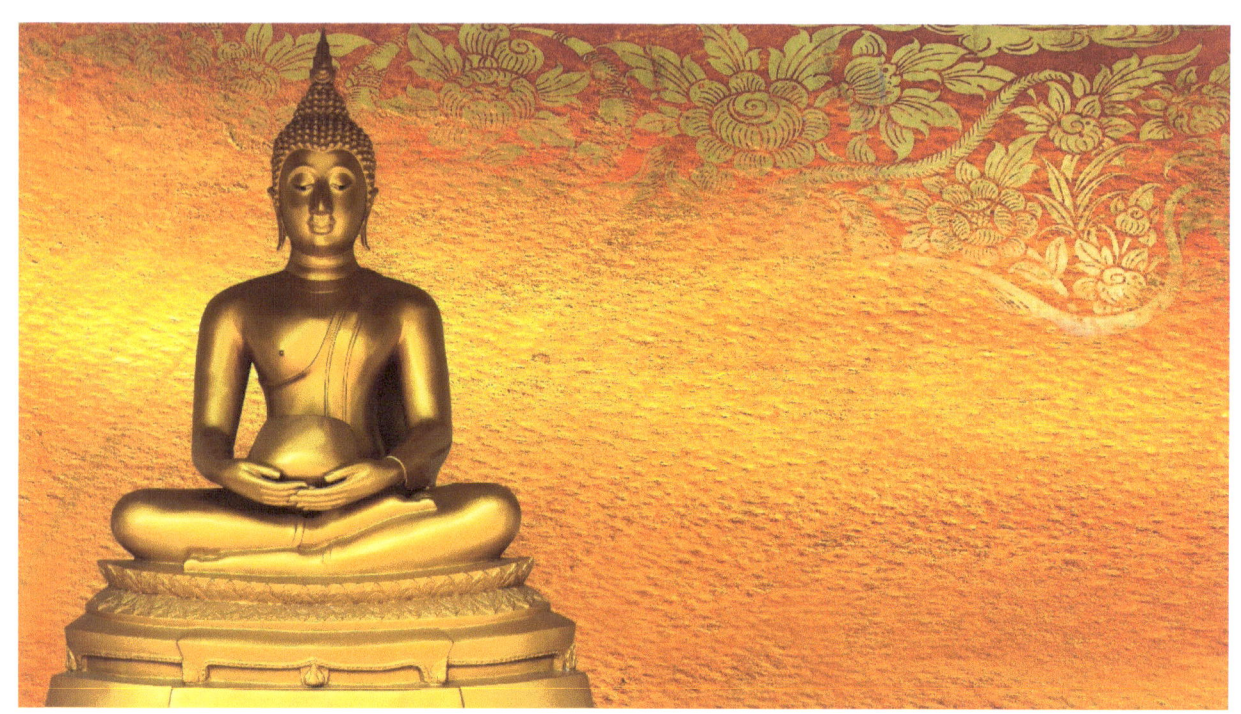

IT IS THE MARK OF AN EDUCATED

MIND TO ENERTAIN A THOUGHT

WITHOUT EXCEPTING IT!

ARISTOTLE

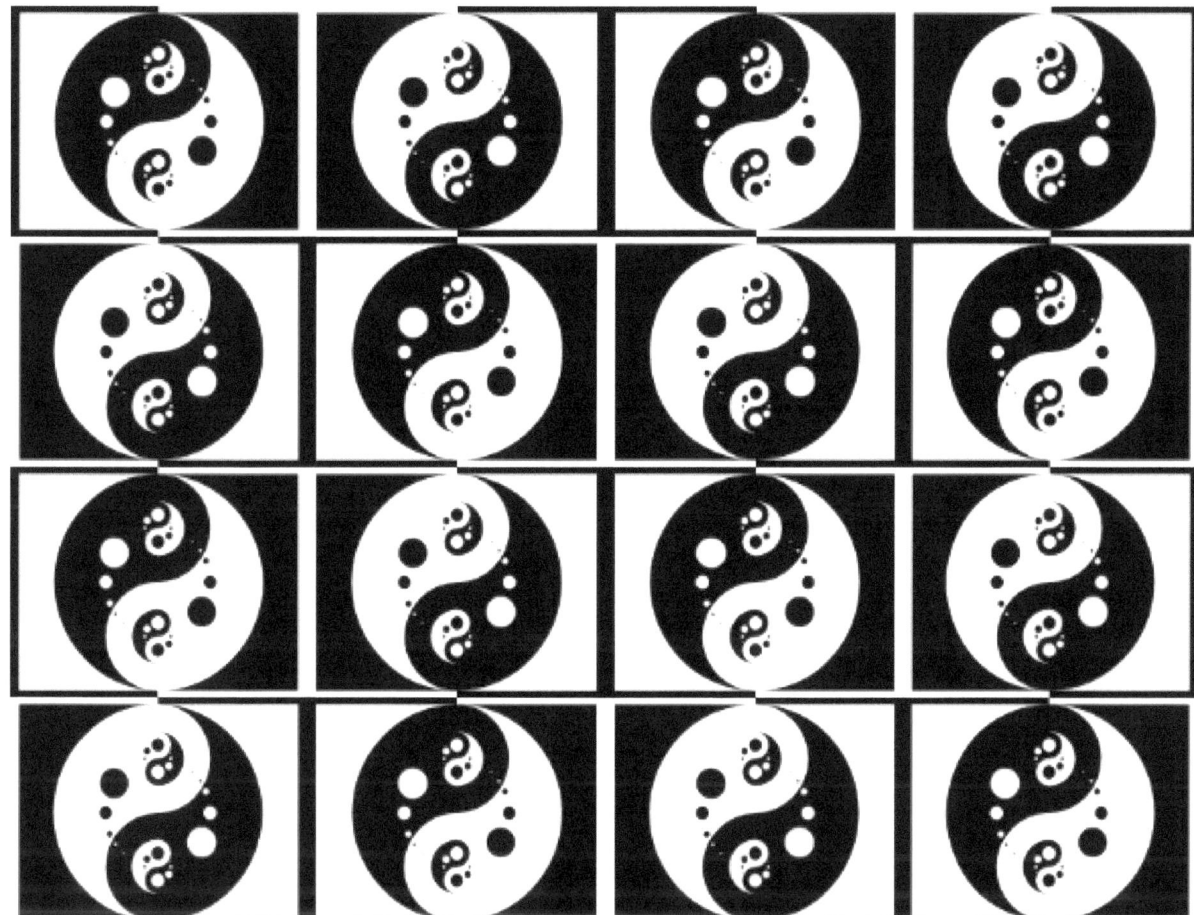

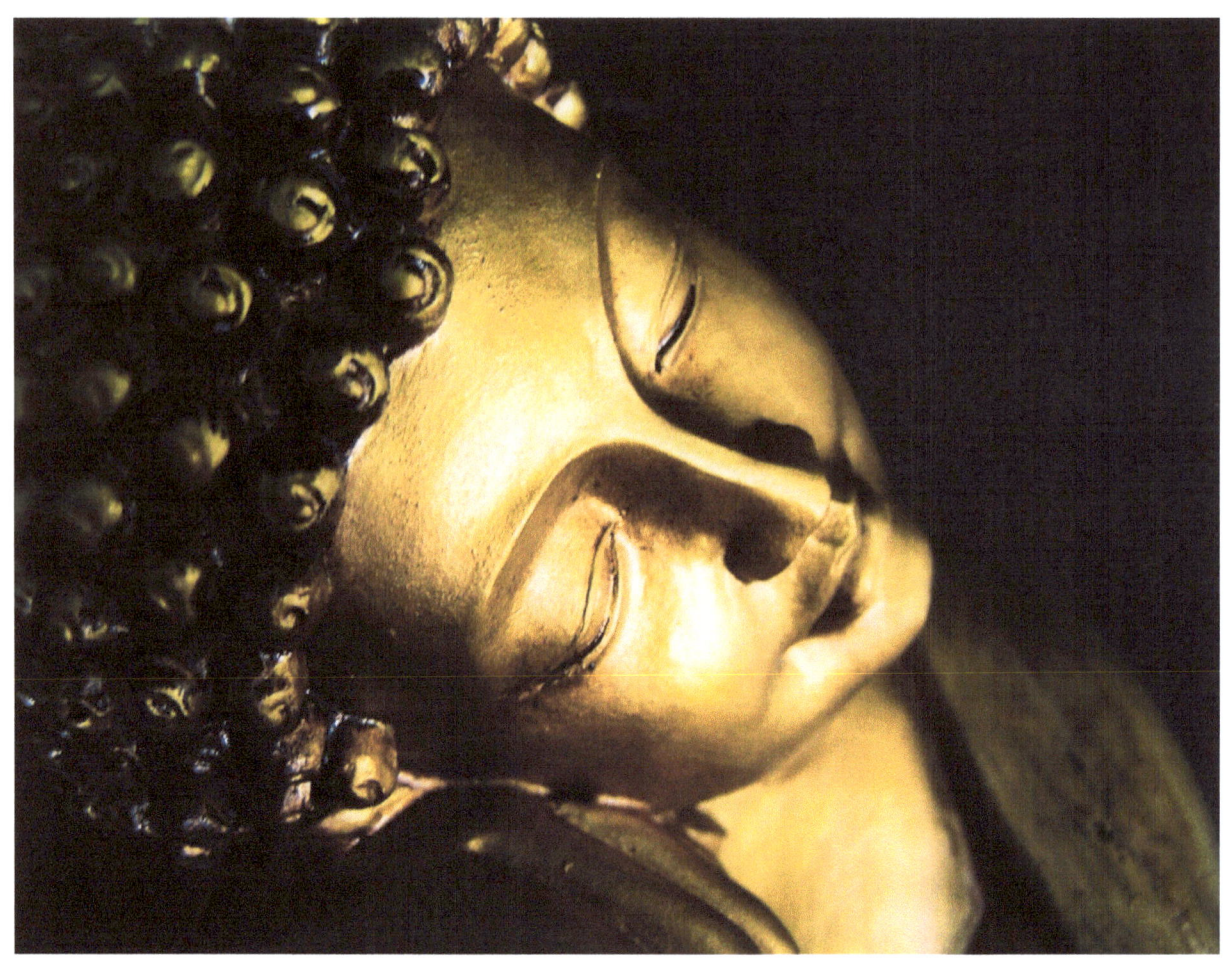

EDUCATION IS THE MOST POWERFUL

WEAPON, WHICH YOU CAN USE

TO CHANGE THE WORLD!

NELSON MANDELA

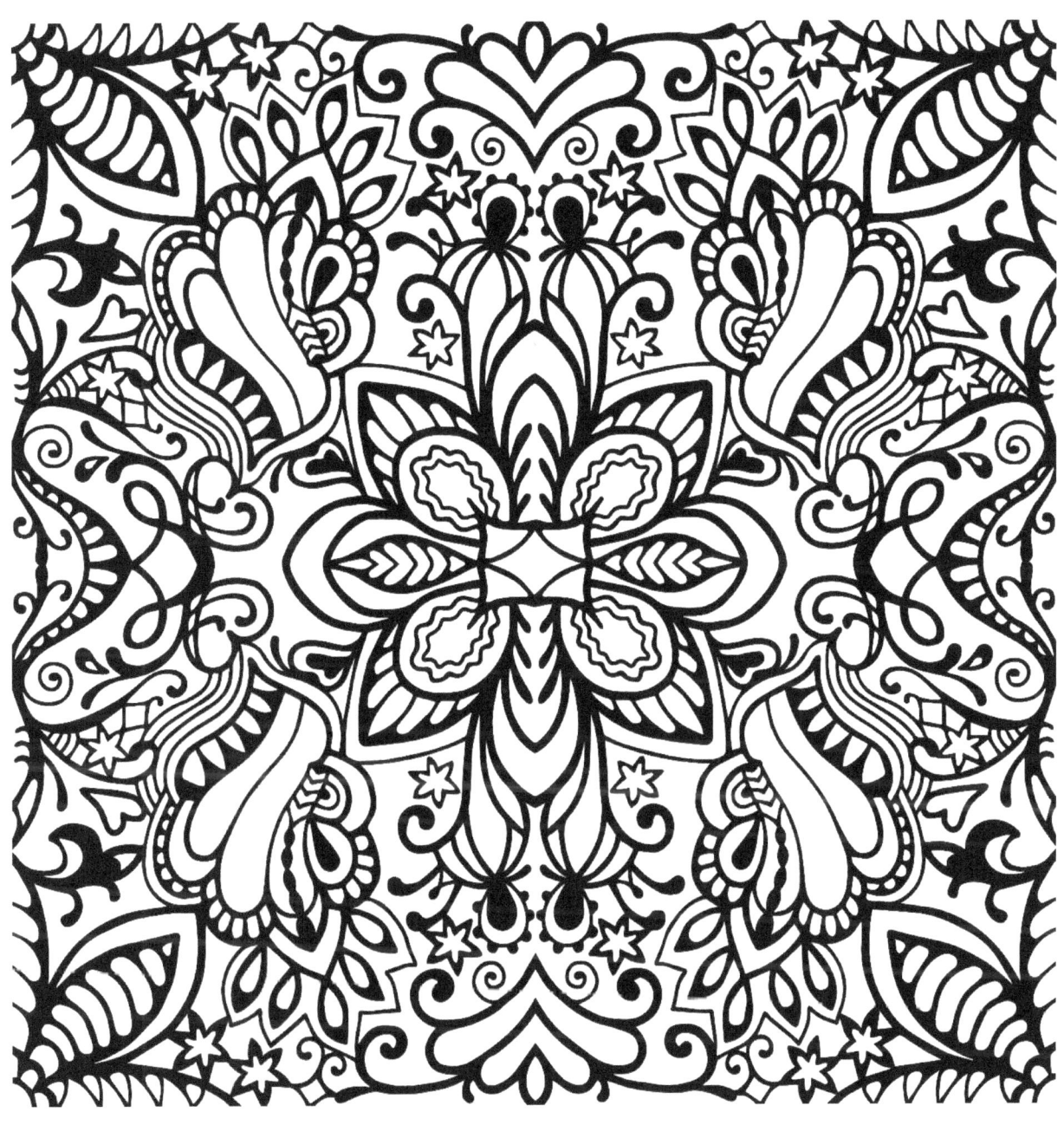

THANK YOU FOR PURCHASING

THIS MANDALA MEDITATION COLORING BOOK!

IF YOU LIKE THIS BOOK AND WOULD

LIKE TO COLOR MORE,

BE SURE TO CHECK OUT OUR

INTERMEDIATE & ADVANCED LEVEL

MANDALA MEDITATION COLORING BOOKS!

CHECK US OUT AT:

WWW.CELESTIALAZUL.COM

OR ON OUR YOUTUBE CHANNEL

WHERE WE HAVE MEDITATIONAL VIDEOS

TO HELP DEEPEN YOUR EXPERIENCE IN MEDITATION!

NAMASTE!